Published By Robert Corbin

@ George Harris

Go Vegan 2023: Benefits of a Vegan Lifestyle and

Tasty Vegan Recipes

All Right RESERVED

ISBN 978-1-7385954-7-1

TABLE OF CONTENTS

Black Beans Soup

Ingredients:

- 1 Teaspoon of dried oregano

- 1/8 Teaspoon of cayenne pepper

- 1 Pinch of freshly ground black pepper

- ½ lb of undrained organic black beans

- ¼ Can of organic tomato sauce

- ¾ Cup of water

- 1 Teaspoon of olive oil

- 1 White chopped onion

- 3 Minced garlic cloves

- 1 and ½ tablespoons of chili powder

- 2 Teaspoons of cumin

Directions:

1. Heat the olive oil into a large saucepan over a medium heat and once the oil gets hot, add in the onions and the garlic and stir for 5 minutes
2. Add the chili powder, the cumin, the oregano, the cayenne pepper and the black pepper.
3. Add the black beans, the tomato sauce and the water; make sure not to drain the black beans
4. Let the soup boil on a low heat for about 25 minutes; then adjust the seasoning with salt
5. Garnish with cilantro; then serve and enjoy with tortilla chip!

Lentil Salad

Ingredients:

- 1 Chopped carrot stick

- ¼ of a small chopped cucumber

- 1 Medium thinly sliced radish

- ¼ Cup of chopped dates

- 2 Tablespoons of toasted sunflower seeds

- 2 tablespoons of olive oil

- 2 tablespoons of balsamic vinegar

- 1 tablespoon of Dijon mustard

- 1 tablespoon of maple syrup

- 1/3 Cup of dry green lentils

- 1 Chopped Wheat pita pocket

- 2 Teaspoons of olive oil

- 2 Teaspoons of rosemary

- 4 Cups of loosely packed arugula

- 2 Chopped celery stalks

Directions:

1. To prepare the maple Dijon vinaigrette
2. Whisk your INGREDIENTS: altogether and set it aside.
3. To prepare the lentil Fattoush salad:
4. Combine the lentils with 2/3 cup of water into a medium sized pot and set it aside to boil on a low heat for about 35 minutes
5. Drain the lentils and let it cool for 5 minutes; then preheat your oven to about 425° F.
6. Toss the pita pieces with the olive oil and the rosemary; sprinkle sea salt; then spread the pita on a cookie sheet lined with a parchment paper and bake it for about 7 minutes

7. Mix the arugula, the lentils, the veggies, the dates, the sunflower seeds, and the pita croutons.

8. Toss your salad with the prepared dressing and divide it between 3 bowls.

9. Serve and enjoy your salad!

Light Lentil Salad

Ingredients:

- 1/2 teaspoon paprika, preferably smoked

- 1/4 teaspoon salt

- 1/4 teaspoon freshly ground pepper

- 2 cups cooked brown rice

- 1 15-ounce can lentils, rinsed, or 11/3 cups cooked lentils

- 1 carrot, diced

- 2 tablespoons chopped fresh parsley

- 2 tablespoons extra-virgin olive oil

- 2 tablespoons sherry vinegar or red-wine vinegar

- 1 tablespoon finely chopped shallot

- 1 tablespoon Dijon mustard

Directions:

1. Whisk oil, vinegar, shallot, mustard, paprika, salt and pepper in a large bowl.
2. Add rice, lentils, carrot and parsley; stir to combine.

Vegan Baked Beans

Ingredients:

- 1 Tablespoon organic Tamari (or other soy sauce)

- 2 to 3 teaspoons minced canned chipotle chilies

- 6 cups cooked Great Northern beans, or 4 (15 oz) cans Great Northern beans, drained and rinsed well

- 1 1/4 cups barbecue sauce

- 3/4 cup dark beer

- 3 Tablespoons dijon mustard

- 3 Tablespoons (packed) organic dark brown sugar

- 6 slices Fakin' bacon (tempeh bacon strips), or other vegetarian bacon*

- 2 Tablespoons extra-virgin olive oil

- 1 1/2 cup chopped onions

- 2 Tablespoons vegetarian Worcestershire sauce

Directions:

1. Preheat oven to 350F.
2. Cook bacon in a swipe of olive oil in a large skillet over medium heat until crisp. Let cool.
3. Pour olive oil into a bowl. Crumble crisped "bacon" into bowl.
4. Add onion, BBQ sauce, beer, mustard, brown sugar, Worcestershire sauce and Tamari and whisk to blend.
5. Add 2-4 teaspoons chipotles, depending on the spiciness desired. Stir in beans.

6. Transfer bean mixture to a lightly oiled 9x13 glass baking dish.

7. Bake uncovered until liquid bubbles and thickens slightly, about 45 minutes. Cool 10 minutes. Serve.

Vegan Quinoa Pizza

Ingredients:

- Sea salt to taste

- 1 cup fire roasted tomato sauce for topping

- 1 cup shredded vegan chees for topping

- 1 tbsp. vegan meat crumbles for topping

- 1 cup of mix veggies chopped for topping (desired)

- 2 tbsp. chopped basil for topping

- ¾ cup quinoa (soaked overnight and drained)

- ¼ cup roasted red pepper humus

- 1-2 tbsp. water

- 1 tsp. baking powder

- Roasted red pepper flakes for topping

Directions:

1. Preheat oven to 425° F.
2. Add all INGREDIENTS: in a food processor and process it until smooth and creamy.
3. Spread it on round lined baking sheet
4. Bake it for 15-20 minutes.
5. Now top it with toppings.
6. Then bake it for additional 10 minutes.
7. Serve hot!

Vegan Stuffed Sweet Potato

Ingredients:

- 1 cup kale chopped

- ½ cup hazelnuts toasted

- 1-2 cloves garlic grated

- ½ tbsp. lemon juice

- Salt and pepper to taste

- 1tbsp. tahini for garnishing

- 2 sweet potatoes (baked)

- 1 cup quinoa(cooked)

- 1 tbsp. olive oil

- 1 red onion chopped

Directions:

1. Heat oil in a pan; saute garlic and onions.

2. Add remaining INGREDIENTS: except sweet potato and cook it for 5 minutes.

3. Turn off the flame and allow it to cool

4. Split the potatoes from center and open it.

5. Now stuff it with prepared mixture.

6. Garnish it with tahini and enjoy!

Veggie Spring Rolls

INGREDIENTS:

For spring rolls:

- 1 cup carrot, grated

- 4 rice paper wrappers

- 4large fresh mint leaves

- 4 large fresh basil

- 1 small beet, halved, thinly sliced

- 1 small ripe avocado, peeled, thinly sliced

- 1 small radish, peeled, thinly sliced

- 1 cup red cabbage, finely chopped

For peanut sauce:

- A pinch crushed red pepper

- 1 tablespoon tamari or soy sauce

- 1 teaspoon rice vinegar

- 1 clove garlic, minced

- 2 tablespoons natural peanut butter

- 1 tablespoon water

- 2 teaspoons pure maple syrup

Directions:

1. Take a shallow dish and pour very hot water in it.
2. Dip 2 rice wrapper in it and let it soak for about 30 seconds or until soft.
3. Gently remove from the bowl and shake to drop off excess water. Place on your cutting board.
4. Repeat with the remaining wrappers.

5. Divide and place beets, avocado and radish next to each other (in the same order given) on the center of the wrappers.
6. Place carrots on top of the beets and cabbage on top of the avocado and radish.
7. Place a basil leaf on the carrot and a mint leaf on the cabbage.
8. Fold over the filling and wrap tightly like a burrito. Cut into 2 halves.
9. Serve with the peanut sauce.
10. To make sauce: Mix together all the INGREDIENTS: of the sauceintoa bowl until smooth and well combined.

Cauliflower And Chickpea Stew With Couscous

INGREDIENTS:

- 2 cans (28 ounces each) whole tomatoes

- 1 teaspoon ground ginger

- 3 teaspoons ground cumin

- Salt to taste

- Pepper to taste

- 1 cup raisins

- 2 cups couscous

- Hot water, as required

- 4 tablespoons olive oil

- 2 heads cauliflower, cut into small florets

- 2 medium onions, chopped

- 10 ounces baby spinach

- 2 cans (15 ounces each) chickpeas, rinsed

Directions:

1. Place a large saucepan over medium heat.
2. Add oil. When oil is heated, add onions and garlic and sauté until the onions are translucent.
3. Add spices and salt and sauté for a few seconds until fragrant.
4. Crush the tomatoes and add into the saucepan.
5. Add rest of the INGREDIENTS: except couscous and spinach. Add about 1 cup water.
6. Simmer until cauliflower is tender and the stew thickened.
7. Add spinach and cook until it wilts. Remove from heat.

8. Add couscous into a large bowl. Pour about 2 cups of hot water over it.

9. Cover and set aside for 5-6 minutes. Take a fork and fluff the couscous.

10. Serve stew with couscous.

Breakfast Hummus Toast

Ingredients:

- 1 tbsp hemp seeds

- 1 tbsp sunflower seeds, unsalted, roasted

- ¼ cup hummus

- 2 slices wheat bread, sprouted, toasted

Directions:

1. Top the toasted bread with hummus, sunflower seeds and hemp seeds. Serve and enjoy!

Almond Milk Banana Smoothie

Ingredients:

- 2 bananas, frozen

- 2 tbsps cacao powder

- ¾ cup almond milk

- 2 tbsps peanut butter

For topping:

- ½ banana, dashed

- Chocolate granola

Directions:

1. Blend cacao powder, bananas, almond milk, peanut butter and in a blender until smooth.
2. Transfer to a bowl and top with sliced banana and granola.

Enjoy and serve.

Vegan Chickpea Curry Coat Potatoes

Ingredients:

- 1 1/2 tsp cumin seeds

- 1 green chilli, finely chopped

- 1/2 tsp turmeric

- 1 big onion, diced

- 2 garlic cloves, crushed

- 2 x 400g can chickpeas, drained

- Lemon wedges and coriander leaves, for garnish

- 2 tbsp tikka masala paste

- 1 tsp ground coriander

- 4 sweet potatoes

- 1 tbsp coconut oil

- 2 x 400g can chopped tomatoes

- 1 tsp garam masala

- Thumb-sized bit ginger, well grated

Directions:

1. Heat the oven to 200c. Pierce the sweet potatoes with a fork, then place them on a baking sheet and roast in the oven for 45 minutes or until tender when pierced with a knife.
2. Melt coconut oil in a large saucepan over medium heat.
3. Add the cumin seeds and fry for 1 minute until they are aromatic, then add the onion and simmer for 7-10 minutes until they soften.

4. Place the ginger, garlic and green chilli in the pan and cook for 2-3 minutes.
5. Add the spices and tikka masala pasta and cook for another 2 minutes until aromatic, then add the berries.
6. Bring to a simmer, then put the chickpeas and cook for 20 more minutes until it thickens.
7. Place roasted sweet potatoes on four plates and then open them lengthwise.
8. Spoon inside the chickpea curry and then squeeze the lemon slices.
9. Season, then spread the coriander before serving.

Vegan Caronia

Ingredients:

Pasta

- 1 cup chopped Portobello mushroom

- 1 cup pre-cooked VEGAN bacon chopped into 1 inch squares (omit if unavailable)

- 1 cup cashews (soaked for at least an hour)

- 1 ½ cup plant milk

- ½ cup nutritional yeast ¼ cup pasta water
  Seasonings:

- Salt

- Pepper

- Crushed red pepper

- Garlic powder

- Onion powder

Directions:

1. Boil pasta and drain. Set aside small amount of pasta water for sauce. In a food processor OR blender blend cashews, nutritional yeast, garlic powder, onion powder and plant milk until smooth.
2. Add salt and pepper and taste. Adjust seasoning as necessary.
3. Next in a large pan, sauté mushrooms and VEGAN bacon in oil.
4. Add pasta, cashew sauce and pasta water.
5. Toss and top with crushed red pepper before serving.

Mushroom Mac And Cheese

INGREDIENTS:

- Boiled elbow macaroni

- 1 cup mushroom

- 1 potato and 1 carrot BOILED and chopped

- 1 ½ cups plant milk

- 1 cup nutritional yeast ¼ cup vegetable stock
  Seasonings:

- 2 tsp Garlic powder

- 2 tsp Onion powder

- Salt

- Pepper

- 2 tsp Paprika

- ½ tsp chilli powder 1 tbsp olive oil

Directions:

1. In a blender or food processor blend boiled potatoes and carrots, plant milk, nutritional yeast, veggie stock, garlic/onion powder, paprika and chilli powder until smooth.
2. Add salt and pepper to taste, and set cheese sauce aside.
3. In a nonstick pot, sauté mushrooms in olive oil until tender.
4. Combine macaroni, cheese sauce and mushroom over low heat and stir. Add salt & pepper to taste.

Cranberry Cabbage

Ingredients:

- A quarter tsp. of ground cloves

- 10 ounces/283 g of canned whole-berry cranberry sauce

- 2 tbsp. of fresh lemon juice

- 2 medium head red cabbage

Directions:

1. You need a large pan to cook the cranberry cabbage.

2. To the pan, add the cranberry sauce, cloves, and lemon juice. Heat them. Once they are heated, simmer them on the stove. The sauce should melt completely.

3. To this melted sauce, add the red cabbage. Stir the INGREDIENTS: well to mix completely.

4. Make the mixture to boil. At this stage, reduce the heat to simmer.
5. Cook for a few minutes and the cabbage should turn soft. Keep stirring.
6. Serve the cranberry cabbage immediately or store for later.

Orange Chickpea Tofu Bowls

Ingredients:

- 3 tsps. of sesame oil (use any oil that you may like)

- 2 (about 14 ounces/ 396 g) package of tofu (slice into cubes)

- A cup of rice

- Green onion and sesame seeds for topping (optional)

- 2 tbsp. of sodium (low) tamari

- 2 (about 15 ounces/ 425g) can of chickpeas (drain the chickpeas and rinse them)

- 7 cups of broccoli

For the orange sauce,

- A half-cup of orange juice (prefer freshly squeezed juice)

- 3 tsps. of cornstarch

- 2 clove of garlic (grated)

- A quarter cup of water

- Half a tsp. of ginger (fresh and grated)

- 3 tbsps. each of

- Tamari of low sodium

- Maple syrup (pure)

- Sesame oil (toasted)

Directions:

1. Cook the rice as per the Directions: given in the packet.
2. Boil the broccoli in water until it reaches the tenderness of desire.

3. Add all the INGREDIENTS: (instructed for preparing the orange juice), in a small-sized bowl (or a jar). Mix them properly to combine.

4. Put the flame of your oven to heat (medium) and place a skillet (large-sized) on it.

5. Add 3 tsp of cooking oil (you prefer) to skillet and allow the oil to come to boil.

6. Now add 2 tbsp. of tamari and tofu to the oil and blend until the tofu gives a brown color. It will just take ten minutes to give out this color on stirring.

7. Add orange juice and chickpeas to the pan and let it boil until the orange sauce becomes condensed.

8. If you are not a person who likes thickened sauce, just make a less diluted 2 by adding more sauce!

9. Directions: of the bowls: add half a cup of rice (heaping), a quarter of the orange tofu, a

quarter of broccoli and chickpeas (cooked) to each bowl.

10. Tamari or soy sauce will be a splendid choice to season the chickpea bowls.

11. Garnish with drizzled sauce and enjoy.

Sweet Potato Salad

Ingredients:

- 1 diced shallot

- 2 finely cut spring onions

- 1 small bunch of chopped chives

- 3 tablespoons of wine vinegar

- 2 teaspoons of olive oil

- 1 tablespoon of pure maple syrup

- 1 pinch of salt

- 2 large peeled and diced sweet potatoes

- 1 tablespoon of olive oil

- ½ teaspoon of paprika, cayenne pepper and oregano

- 1 pinch of ground black pepper

Directions:

1. Preheat your oven to about 390°F; then line a baking sheet with a parchment paper.
2. Toss the sweet potato chunks with 1 to 2 tablespoons of extra virgin olive oil and add the optional spices.
3. Spread the potato chunks on the lined baking sheet and bake it in your oven for about 35 minutes until it is perfectly roasted.
4. Remove the sweet potatoes from the oven and set it aside to cool
5. Prepare your dressing by mixing the shallots, the scallions, the chives, the vinegar, the olive oil, and the maple syrup.
6. Toss the sweet potatoes with the dressing and garnish with topping of your choice like chives
7. Refrigerate the salad for about an hour; then serve and enjoy it!

Kale Salad

Ingredients:

- 2 medium bell peppers

- 1 medium sized green zucchini

- 1 and ½ cups of cooked chilled quinoa

- 1 cup of cooked rinsed and drained chickpeas

- 1 sliced avocado

- 1 thinly sliced red onion

- 2 sliced portabella mushrooms

- 2 teaspoons of sunflower oil

- 2 tablespoons of balsamic vinegar

- 2lb of asparagus

- 1 finely chopped kale head

- 3 cups of chopped cabbage

- 3 small radishes

Directions:

1. Prepare your dressing first; then trim the ends of the asparagus and chop it into chunks of small size.
2. Steam the asparagus for about 7 minutes and after that; drain it and pat dry it.
3. To cook the mushrooms; place it into a small pan and add a little bit of oil; then cook it for about 3 minutes. Once it becomes hot; add 2 tbsp of balsamic vinegar and cook for 6 minutes
4. Let the mushroom cool for about 5 minutes; then slice and chop the pepper, the zucchini and the radish.
5. Put the kale and the cabbage into a large mixing bowl and then toss it with the desired amount of dressing it needs

6. Add the asparagus, the radishes, the pepper, the zucchini, the quinoa, and the chickpeas into a bowl; then toss it with the greens and add more dressing if you need more.

7. Serve your salad into large bowls with the cooled mushrooms, the sliced avocado, the sliced red onion, the pepper; the sesame seeds.

8. Enjoy a tasty salad!

Vegan Jamaican Curry

Ingredients:

- ½ cup asparagus

- ½ cup tender stem broccoli chopped

- ¾ cup chickpeas (cooked)

- 1 cup coconut milk

- Water as needed

- 1 bay leaf

- 1 tbsp. dried thyme

- 1 tsp. ginger powder

- 1 tbsp. Jamaican curry powder or to taste

- Salt and black pepper to taste

- 1 tbsp. olive oil

- 3 garlic cloves grated

- ½ scotch bonnet chopped

- ¼ cup tomato puree

- 1 cup spring onions chopped

- 1 red pepper chopped

- 1 cup zucchini chopped

- ½ cup beans chopped

Directions:

1. Heat oil in a pan; saute garlic and onions.
2. Add all spices and cook it for 2-3 minutes.
3. Now add veggies and cook it for 5 minutes.
4. Add remaining INGREDIENTS: and mix it well.
5. Simmer it for 10 -15 min.
6. Garnish it with coconut flakes and enjoy!

Vegan Pad Thai

Ingredients:

- 2 tbsp. tamarind sauce

- 1 tbsp. raw sugar

- 1 tbsp. rice vinegar

- 1 tbsp. sriracha sauce

- ½ tbsp. lemon juice

- 2-3 rice noodles(soaked in warm water,10-15 min and drained)

- 1 ½ cup tofu (cooked - crispy)

- Handful bean sprout for garnishing

- 1 tbsp. olive oil

- 3-4 garlic cloves grated

- 1 red chili chopped

- 1 shallot chopped

- 2 green onions chopped

- 3-4 cup vegetables julienned (desired)

- ¼ cup soy sauce

Directions:

1. Heat oil in a pan; add garlic, onions, shallots, red chili and cook it for 2-3 min.
2. Now add all veggies and cook it for 5-8 min.
3. Then add all sauces, vinegar and lemon juice.
4. Mix it well, now add noodles and tofu.
5. Cook it for additional 2-3 minutes.
6. Serve it with bean sprout.

Vegan Red Lentil Dal

Ingredients:

- Half a tsp. of pepper and salt

- 3 tsps. of turmeric

- 2 15 ounces/425 g can coconut milk (light or fat-free)

- Three cups of water

- 2 tsp. each of:

- Ginger

- Cumin

- 2 tbsp. of curry powder

- 3 cups of red lentils (dried)

Directions:

1. Set a pot full of water on the oven so it starts to boil.
2. Add coconut milk and lentils to the boiling water.
3. Continue boiling and let it simmer. Cook the mixture for about ten minutes and allow the lentils to soften down.
4. Add the spices and cook for about five minutes.
5. Serve the dish with cauliflower rice, flatbreads, brown or white rice or quinoa, and enjoy with your family.

Vegan Sun-Dried Tomato Meatballs

Ingredients:

For the chickpea meatballs

- Freshly chopped basil (packed loosely)

- Bread crumbs, panko (GF eaters must consume the gluten-free 2)

- Chopped tomatoes, sun dried (packed loosely)

- 3 tablespoons of olive oil

- Optional-2 tablespoon of oregano, dried (3 tablespoons of fresh oregano, chopped per 2 tablespoon dried)

- 2 batch of flax egg (2 tablespoon of flaxseed meal plus 3-and-a-half tablespoon of water)

- 2 15 oz./425 g can of chickpeas (it should be dried, drained and rinsed)

- 2 pinch of pepper flakes (red) and sea salt

- Three cloves of garlic (minced)

- 2-third cup each of

- Parmesan cheese (vegan)

For the coating

- Three tablespoons of bread crumbs, panko

- 3 tablespoons of parmesan cheese (vegan)

Directions:

1. Keep your oven heated by setting its temperature at 375 degrees Fahrenheit/190 degrees Celsius.

2. Place a large-sized skillet (made of iron or metal) on top of the oven. Once the skillet is warm, add the garlic (minced) and half of the olive oil, as menti2d in the recipe INGREDIENTS: (adjust with altering batches).

Stir this mixture for about three minutes. This period will be enough to turn the garlic light brown. After you are d2, keep it off the oven and let it cool.

3. In a high-speed blender, prepare the flaxseed meal as per directed in the recipe INGREDIENTS:. Once it is properly blended, add the oil-garlic mixture into the blender.

4. To the blender add basil, parmesan cheese (vegan), pepper flakes, 2 tablespoon of olive oil, salt, tomatoes (sun-dried), and bread crumbs 2 after the other and pulse these INGREDIENTS:. Pulse until it forms tiny particles. Scrape sides of the blender using a scraper.

5. Add the chickpeas (drain with water and rinse before using) and blend them into the blender. Blend until the mixture forms dough enough to make putty in hands. The chickpeas

should neither be a paste nor should have any whole piece. It should be intermediate.

6. Adjust the INGREDIENTS: for seasoning as you would like to have it.

7. Prepare a parmesan cheese-bread crumb mixture on a plate. Scoop out 2 tablespoon amount of dough and circle them into balls (approximately 15 balls). And coat the balls with the cheese-bread crumbs mixture.

8. Heat the same skillet you have been using by turning the flame to medium heat and pour 3 tablespoons of olive oil to its base to form a layer that is thin. Add the meatballs 2 by 2, try not to crowd the pan, and therefore add in batches. More oil is to be added if needed.

9. Simmer the oven and toss the pan to circle the balls for about 5 minutes. This will help to cook the meatballs evenly on all the sides without browning them too much.

10. Place the tomato meatballs on the baking sheet. Bake them for 15 minutes. Cook the meatballs till golden brown and make sure its texture becomes firm before taking it off the oven. The longer they will cool, the more they will firm up.

11. In the meantime, you can prepare any sauce you like to have with the meatballs, but the marinara sauce would be the best to go with. Prepare the pasta as well for a side dish.

12. Serve the pasta with marinara sauce and the number of meatballs as you want to have at a time because there are storing options too!

13. Sprinkle some more cheese (shredded) and basil.

Vegan Breakfast Sandwich

Ingredients:

- 1/2 teaspoon garlic powder

- ¼ teaspoon ground black pepper

- 1/2 teaspoon black salt

- 1 teaspoon turmeric

- 1 tablespoon coconut oil

- 2 tablespoons vegan mayo

- 3 slices of vegan cheese

- 1 cup of spinach

- 6 slices of pickle

- 14 oz tofu , extra-firm, pressed

- 2 medium tomatoes , sliced

- 6 slices of gluten-free bread, toasted

Directions:

1. Cut tofu into 7 slices, and then season its 2 side with garlic, black pepper, salt, and turmeric.
2. Take a skillet pan, place it over medium heat, add oil and when hot, add seas2d tofu slices in it, season side down, and cook for 3 minutes until crispy and light brown.
3. Then flip the tofu slices and continue cooking for 3 minutes until browned and crispy.
4. When d2, transfer tofu slices on a baking sheet, in the form of a set of 3 slices side by side, then top each set with a cheese slice and broil for 3 minutes until cheese has melted.
5. Spread mayonnaise on both sides of slices, top with 3 slices of tofu, cheese on the side, top with spinach, tomatoes, pickles, and then close the sandwich.
6. Cut the sandwich into half and then serve.

Vegan Fried Egg

Ingredients:

- ½ teaspoon ground black pepper

- ½ teaspoon salt

- 1 tablespoon vegan butter

- 1 block of firm tofu, firm, pressed, drained

- 1 cup vegan toast dipping sauce

Directions:

1. Cut tofu into four slices, and then shape them into a rough circle by using a cookie cutter.
2. Take a frying pan, place it over medium heat, add butter and when it melts, add prepared tofu slices in a single layer and cook for 3 minutes per side until light brown.
3. Transfer tofu to serving dishes, make a small hole in the middle of tofu by using a small

cookie cutter and fill the hole with dipping sauce.

4. Garnish eggs with black pepper and sauce and then serve.

Collard Green Spring Rolls

Ingredients:

For the spring rolls

- 10 oz./283 g of tofu (for better taste circle in sesame and brush with tamari)

- Three medium-sized carrots, peeled (chopped finely)

- 2 and a half cups of sprouts (bean)

- 2 bundle of collard green (per bundle consisting of eleven to twelve large-sized collards)

- 2 cup each of:

- Red cabbage (sliced finely)

- Basil packed

- 2 small-sized bell pepper (sliced thinly and vertically)

For the sauce

- 2-third cup of creamy sunflower-seed butter (unsalted)

- Warm water

- Half a lime juiced (medium-sized)

- 2 half to 3 tablespoons of tamari (replace with soy sauce if not GF)

- Half a teaspoon of chili-garlic sauce (a quarter teaspoon of pepper flakes, red would also do)

- 2-3 tablespoons of maple syrup

Directions:

1. Wrap up the tofu with a towel that can absorb the water well from it. It has to be a clean 2. Place something heavy on the top of the

wrapped tofu. This will help to drain out excess water from the tofu.

2. While you are allowing the tofu to drain the moisture, use this time to prepare the collard greens. Chop off the stems of collard with the help of a small and sharp knife. Chopping off means to just trim the width of stems only at the foot of each leaf. It will only allow the collards to fold in easily while making the rolls.

3. Now you need to prepare the vegetables and cut the tofu into slices. Make the tofu into rectangular cubes and arrange the cubes on a cutting board by slightly dampening the central portion of the cutting board.

4. Use a small-sized mixing bowl to prepare the dipping sauce. Add tamari, lime juice, sunflower seed butter, maple syrup, and chili-garlic sauce to the bowl. Whip all the INGREDIENTS: together to combine well.

Dilute the sauce by adding warm water to it until it becomes a semi-thick fluid. Make it so thick that it can be poured. Adjust the taste and flavor according to your desire by adding more lime juice, chili-garlic sauce, maple syrup and tamari for acidity, heat, sweetness, and saltiness respectively.

5. Lay down the collard green on a flat surface. Start laying the INGREDIENTS: (to prepare the filling) at the stem of the collards. The INGREDIENTS: include basil, red pepper, bean sprout, tofu, cabbage, and carrot. Bend over the collards to keep the veggies secured inside it and turn the sides of collards inwards. Continue to roll down the sides of collards until you get a loose-spring roll. You can do this with your hands. Make the use of all the veggies by making the number of rolls you desire to have.

6. Take a serving plate and place the rolls so that the seam-side faces the plate.

7. You will get 11-12 spring rolls with the INGREDIENTS: menti2d in the recipe.

8. The number of rolls can increase depending on the batch size.

9. Serve the rolls with the dipping sauce poured over them. Enjoy the warm and delicious rolls immediately.

Chickpea Curry

Ingredients:

- Half tsp. of chili flakes

- 3 cloves of garlic (Minced)

- 10 ounces/283 g of fresh baby spinach (Uncooked) - ten cups of loosely packed spinach, or 10 ounces/283 g frozen spinach

- Four wedges of lemon (optional)

- 2 tsp. of olive oil

- Fresh coriander (optional)

- 3 tsps. of turmeric

- Salt to taste

- 2 can of coconut milk

- 2 tsp. of ginger powder

- 2 medium-sized onion (Chopped)

- 3 tsps. of garam masala

- 3 cans of chickpeas fifteen oz./425 g per can (Rinsed and drained)

Directions:

1. Start with heating the oil. Use a large pan for this. When the oil is smoking hot, bring the flame down. Add ginger powder, chili flakes, garam masala, and turmeric.
2. Toss for a few seconds and add the minced garlic and chopped onions.
3. Onions and garlic will turn brown in a minute, and after that, pour the coconut milk, and add the chickpeas. Add salt to suit your preference.

4. Let the contents cook for 5 minutes. Stir after adding the spinach and cover the pan with a lid.
5. Wait for 2-3 minutes to let the spinach wilt. Now, the chickpea curry is ready to serve.
6. Dash a few drops of lemon juice, freshly squeezed. Use chopped fresh coriander for garnishing, if you prefer. This is however, optional.
7. The chickpea curry suits best with basmati rice or can be spread on naan bread.

Red Beans And Rice

INGREDIENTS:

- 2 cans red kidney beans

- 1 cup green onion (chopped)

- 1 small yellow onion (chopped)

- 1 small green bell pepper (chopped) 3 garlic cloves (minced)

Seasonings:

- Salt & Pepper (to taste)

- 1 tbsp Cayenne

- 2tsp Cumin

- 2tsp Crushed red pepper

Directions:

1. Over medium high heat sauté garlic, yellow onions and bell peppers until tender.
2. Add kidney beans and seasoning, cover and reduce heat to simmer for about 10 minutes. Stir occasionally.
3. Lightly mash some of the bean, add green onion for garnish and place beans over cooked brown rice.

Cucumber Salad

Ingredients:

- ¼ cup fresh parsley and cilantro

- 1 tsp dried oregano

- 1 tsp dried thyme

- 3 tbsp red wine vinegar

- 1 sliced cucumber

- 2 diced roma tomatoes

- ¼ red onion (chopped)

Directions:

1. Toss all INGREDIENTS:, cool in refrigerator and enjoy!

Toasted Chickpeas

Ingredients:

- ½ tsp cinnamon

- ½ tsp sweet paprika

- 6 bread slices, toasted

- ½ tsp sugar

- 2 cup chickpeas, cooked

- ½ tsp salt

- Black pepper, to taste

- 3 small shallots, diced

- 2 large tomatoes, skinned, cho pped

- 2 large garlic cloves, diced

- ¼ tsp smoked paprika

- 2 tbsps olive oil

Directions:

1. Heat olive oil in a pan. Sauté the shallots, frequently stirring until they are almost translucent.
2. Add the garlic and then saute until the garlic softens.
3. Add the spices to the pan. Cook for 1 minute, stirring frequently.
4. Add the tomatoes to the pan. Add a little water, then cook over medium-low heat until a thick sauce forms.
5. Add the chickpeas and cook for 3 minutes, then sprinkle with black pepper, sugar and salt.
6. Cover toasted bread with chickpea mixture and serve.

Almond Milk Chai Quinoa

Ingredients:

- 1 chai tea bag

- ½ cup quinoa, rinsed

- 1 cup almond milk

Directions:

1. Add quinoa, almond milk and chai tea bag in a pan and bring to a boil.
2. Remove the tea bag then reduce the heat. Cook, covered, for 20 minutes.
3. Remove from fire and leave covered 10 minutes.
4. Serve and enjoy.

Savory Vegan Omelet

Ingredients:

For the omelet:

- Olive oil

- 2 garlic cloves, minced

- ¾ cup (5 oz.) Firm tofu, drained, patted dry

- Black pepper and salt

- ¼ tsp paprika

- 2 tbsps nutritional yeast

- 1 tsp cornstarch

For the filling:

- 1 cup veggies (tomato, spinach, etc.), sliced

Directions:

1. Preheat the oven to 375 f.

2. Heat an oven-safe pan over medium heat and then add olive oil and garlic. Cook the garlic for 2 minutes.

3. Add garlic and remaining INGREDIENTS: (except vegetables) to a food processor and mix until smooth and combined. Add 1½ tbsps of water. Set aside.

4. Add more olive oil to the pan. Add the vegetables and sprinkle with pepper and salt. Cook until ready, then reserve.

5. Turn off the heat. Make sure the pan is covered with enough oil. Add ¼ of the vegetables and add the tofu mixture on top.

6. Spread the tofu mixture throughout the pan with a spoon, but do not create spaces in it.

7. Place on the stove and cook over medium heat for 5 minutes. Bake in the oven for 15 minutes. At the 13 minute mark, add the

remaining vegetables on top of the tortilla and cook for an additional 2 minutes.

8. Remove from the oven. Fold with a spatula and serve.

Chili Surprise

Ingredients:

- 3 tbsp chili powder

- pinch sea salt

- pinch cayenne

- 1 can each: black beans, white kidney beans, red kidney beans (rinsed) (I used 1 large mixed can)

- 1 can diced tomatoes with juice

- 2 tsp oregano

- 1 can organic mushrooms, drained

- 1 tbsp unsweetened cocoa powder

- juice of 1 lime (optional, I didn't include)

- Secret Ingredient —> 2 tbsp CHIA SEEDS

- 1 tbsp oil

- 1-3 cloves garlic, minced (I used 1)

- 2 bell peppers, chopped

- 1 sweet onion, chopped

- 3 carrots, chopped

- 1 tbsp cumin

Directions:

1. In a large pot, add the EVOO and heat over medium.
2. dd garlic, peppers, onion, carrot and sauté until everything is soft, approximately 5 minutes.
3. Add the rest of the INGREDIENTS:, cover, and cook for about 30-40 minutes on low to medium heat.

Vegan Brownies

Ingredients:

- 1 cup cake or pastry flour

- 1 cup whole wheat flour

- 3/4 cup dutch process cocoa

- 1 tsp baking powder

- 1 tsp baking soda

- 1 tsp salt

- 2 Tbsp flax seeds (ground)

- 6 Tbsp hot water

- 1 cup coconut oil

- 4 oz. (or 112 grams) bittersweet chocolate

- 1 tsp vanilla

- 2 tsp instant coffee or espresso powder

- 1/2 cup hot water

- 2 cups sugar

Directions:

1. Preheat oven to 350°F and grease an 8 x 8 pan.
2. In a double boiler or a bowl set atop a pot of gently simmering water, melt the coconut oil, chocolate squares and vanilla together.
3. Mix the coffee (or espresso) powder with the 1/2 cup of hot water and stir into the coconut/chocolate mixture.
4. Add sugar and remove from heat.
5. In another bowl, sift together the flours, cocoa, baking powder, baking soda and salt. Whisk to combine.

6. In yet another bowl (small 2), mix the flax seeds and 6 Tbsp of hot water, allow to sit for 2-3 minutes.
7. Combine the chocolate/coconut oil mixture with the flour mixture and stir to incorporate.
8. Add the thickened flax and stir that in as well.
9. Pour the batter into the greased baking pan and bake for 30-40 minutes.
10. When finished, remove the brownies from the oven, set atop a cooling rack.

Beef Chili

Ingredients:

- 3 Garlic cloves (pressed or finely chopped)

- 900 g Beef mince

- 2 tbsp Medium or hot chili powder (to taste)

- 2 tbsp Ground cumin

- 2 tbsp Dried oregano

- 2 tbsp Smoked paprika

- Salt & Pepper to taste

- 500 ml Beef stock

- 50 g Cheddar for topping

- 1 Spring onion (chopped) for topping

- 1 Avocado (smashed) for topping

- 4 slices smoked back bacon (cut into 2cm strips)

- ½ Onion (chopped)

- 2 Celery stalks (chopped)

- 1 Green pepper (deseeded, chopped)

- 50 g Edam cheese or similar (diced)

Directions:

1. In a large frying pan, cook the bacon on a medium heat until crisp and remove. Add the onion and celery to the pan and cook until soft (around 5-6 minutes.) Add the garlic and cook for 1 minute more.

2. Add the beef mince to the pan with the vegetables and cook until browned. Carefully drain away the excess fat and return to the heat.

3. Add the chili powder, cumin, oregano, paprika, salt and pepper. Mix all INGREDIENTS: together to season and cook for a further 2 minutes.

4. Gently stir in the Beef stock and simmer, stirring occasionally for 10-15 minutes until most of the stock has evaporated.

5. Ladle into bowls and top with any remaining crushed bacon, cheese, spring onion and smashed avocado.

Keto Burger Buns

Ingredients:

- 600 g Almond flour

- 2 tbsp Baking soda

- 1 tbsp Salt

- 4 tbsp Butter, melted

- Sesame seeds to taste

- 400g Shredded mozzarella

- 12o g Cream cheese

- 3 Large free-range eggs

- Dried parsley to taste

Directions:

1. Preheat oven to 200°C and line a baking sheet with parchment paper.
2. In a large microwave-safe bowl, melt together mozzarella and cream cheese over 30 second intervals, stirring in between. Careful, the bowl will get hot.
3. Add the eggs and sieve in the almond flour, baking soda and salt to form a neat dough.
4. Separate the dough into 6 balls and gently flatten onto the baking sheet.
5. Brush with the melted butter, top with sesame seeds and parsley.
6. Bake in the centre of the oven until golden. 10-12 minutes

Delicious Florentine Fried Egg Toastie

Ingredients:

- 1 Tablespoon grated cheddar cheese

- 1 small handful of baby spinach

- 1 Tablespoon of olive oil

- 1 large egg

- Hot sauce (any brand)

- 1 scoop of butter

- 2 pieces of white bread

- Watercress or spinach for serving

Directions:

1. With the rim of a glass, make a hole in the center of each slice of bread.

2. Spread the butter onto each slice, pile high with cheese and spinach.
3. Heat the olive oil in a large frying pan over medium heat.
4. Sandwich the bread and use a fish slice to press the bread down into the pan. Cook for 5 minutes until the cheese starts melting.
5. Turn the sandwich over and crack the egg into the hole. Put a lid on top of the pan and cook for 4 minutes.
6. Transfer the sandwich into a plate, drizzle with hot sauce and serve with watercress or spinach on the side.

Tasty Poached Eggs With Tomatoes, Broccoli & Whole Meal Flatbread

Ingredients:

- 2 pieces of whole meal flatbread

- 2 Tablespoons of mixed seeds (pumpkin, sunflower, linseed, sesame)

- 1 Tablespoon of cold pressed rapeseed oil

- A pinch of chili flakes

- ¼ cup broccoli, halved and trimmed

- ¾ cup cherry tomatoes

- 4 large eggs

Directions:

1. Heat the oven to 250 degrees F and warm an ovenproof plate.

2. Boil the kettle and pour the water into a large saucepan a third of the way up and boil over medium heat.

3. Add the broccoli and allow it to cook for 2 minutes.

4. Add the tomatoes and boil for a further 30 seconds.

5. Lift the broccoli and tomatoes out with a slotted spoon and place onto the warm plate.

6. Break the eggs into the water and reduce the temperature to a low heat.

7. Cook for 3 minutes until the yokes are runny and the whites are set.

8. Put the flatbread onto 3 plates, top with the tomatoes and broccoli. Lift the poached eggs out with a slotted spoon and place on top. Sprinkle the seeds over the top and drizzle with oil. Season with the chilli flakes and serve.

Turnip Patties

Ingredients:

- 2 teaspoons of sea salt

- 1 teaspoon of black pepper

- 1 small onion, shredded

- 2 medium or 3 small turnips

- 2 tablespoons of soymilk

- 2 tablespoons of whole wheat flour

Directions:

1. Prepare the turnips by removing the stems and shredding with a large grater into a medium-sized bowl.

2. Using a small grater, shred the onion and combine with the turnip, then stir in the soymilk, flour, sea salt, and black pepper.

87

3. Stir until well mixed, so that the INGREDIENTS: stick together.

4. If needed, add more milk or wheat to thin or thicken the mix. Heat a skillet on medium with olive oil and form 2 patty (3-4 inches in diameter) and fry on each side carefully, to avoid breaking the patty apart.

5. Fry on each side for 3-4 minutes until golden brown, then serve with vegan sour cream and/or salsa or guacamole.

6. Patties can be served on their own with a dash of chili pepper or as a side with a meal.

Vegetarian Shepherd's Pie

Ingredients:

- 1 teaspoon of black pepper

- 1 teaspoon of chili powder

- Dash of sea salt

- 2 large carrots, sliced in small pieces

- 2 stalks of celery, sliced in small pieces

- 1 small onion, diced

- ½ cup of corn

- ½ cup of green peas

- 2 tablespoons of whole wheat flour

- 1 tablespoon of water

- 3-4 tablespoons of soymilk (unflavored, unsweetened)

- 1 cup of uncooked brown lentils

- 1 small package of vegan ground "meat"

- 2 large potatoes

- 2 large sweet potatoes

- 2 cloves of garlic

- 1 teaspoon of fresh dill (or dried)

Directions:

1. Begin this recipe by preheating the oven to 350 degrees and grease a medium to a large baking loaf pan, then set aside.
2. On the stovetop, heat a large skillet with olive oil, and toss in the onion, garlic, and black pepper.

3. Sauté for a few minutes, then add in the vegan ground "meat" and continue to cook.

4. Add in the sea salt and chili powder and continue to cook on medium until brown. If the vegan meat is to be omitted, cook the 2 cup of lentils in 3 cups of boiling water, adding sea salt, then drain and add to the skillet in place of (or in addition to) the ground "meat".

5. When this step is d2, add in the corn, peas, carrots, and celery and continue to fry on medium under vegetables are tender, then gently stir in 3 tablespoons of whole wheat flour, followed by 2 tablespoon of water.

6. Prepare a large casserole dish and grease it lightly.

7. Scoop the vegetable and lentil mix from the skillet and layer the bottom of the dish evenly.

8. To prepare the top layer, mash the yams in a large bowl, add in 3-4 tablespoons of soymilk

and 3 tablespoons of vegan butter and mash together until smooth.

9. Scoop and gently layer over the vegetable mix on the bottom of the dish.

10. Ensure this layer is evenly spread, then top with black pepper, sea salt, and paprika.

11. Bake for 30-35 minutes until the top is slightly golden. Remove and slice to serve.

Vegan Buttermilk Pancakes With Blueberry Sauce

Ingredients:

- Organic, unrefined sugar 1 tablespoon

- All-purpose flour 1 cup

- Zest of 1 lemon

- Baking soda ½ teaspoon

- Baking powder ½ teaspoon

- Pinch of sea salt

- Almond milk 1 cup

- Apple cider vinegar 1 teaspoon

- Medium Banana ½, mashed well

- Vegetable oil 2 tablespoons

93

Directions:

1. Place the almond milk in a bowl, then add apple cider vinegar and let sit until curdled, about 5 to 10 minutes.

2. Pour into a medium-sized mixing bowl and add sugar, vegetable oil, mashed banana and lemon zest. Mix well.

3. Add flour, sea salt, baking powder and baking soda. Whisk until just mix. The mixture will be lumpy and avoid over-mixing.

4. Preheat frying pan to 350F and lightly oil.

5. For each pancake, add ¼ cup batter onto the pan.

6. Cook until bubbles are forming and popping on top, and edges are slightly hardened. Flip over and cook through.

Blueberry Sauce

Ingredients:

- Cinnamon ¼ teaspoon

- Cornstarch or arrowroot powder 1 tablespoon

- Cold water 1 tablespoon

- Unsweetened frozen blueberries 2 cups

- Organic, unrefined sugar 1/3 cup

- Lemon juice 1 tablespoon

- Lemon zest 1 tablespoon

Directions:

1. Add the blueberries, cinnamon, lemon zest, lemon juice, and sugar in a saucepan.
2. Mix cornstarch with cold water in a bowl and mix well.

3. Then whisk into the cinnamon-blueberry mixture and bring to a boil.

4. Lower the heat to a simmer and simmer for a few minutes, or until thickens.

5. Remove from heat and serve.

Vegan Egg Toast With Asparagus

Ingredients:

- Garlic powder ½ teaspoon

- Salt and pepper to taste

- Asparagus Spears 10

- Sourdough bread 2 slices

- Chickpea flour 4 tablespoons

- Nutritional yeast 2 tablespoons

- Black salt 1 teaspoon

Directions:

1. Preheat the grill.
2. In a bowl, mix the chickpea flour with black salt, garlic powder, and nutritional yeast. 2

tablespoon at a time, stir in the water until the mixture is thick but pourable.

3. Evenly spread the flour-yeast mixture onto the bread slices and then arrange the asparagus spears on top.

4. Grill until the chickpea mixture has firmed up and the asparagus is cooked about 8 minutes.

5. Serve.

Cucumber Salad

Ingredients:

- ¼ Cup of parsley

- 1 Medium lemon

- 2 Tbsp of olive oil

- 1 Seedless cucumber

- 2 Ripe firm tomatoes

- ½ Sliced red onion

- ½ of a red pepper

Directions:

1. Finely chop the tomato and the cucumber; then finely chop the pepper.

2. Cut the red onion into very small chunks and finely cut 4 sprigs of parsley.

3. Toss the salad with lemon juice and olive oil.

4. Add the salt and the pepper to taste.

5. Combine your INGREDIENTS: very well; then toss it all together in a bowl and serve it.

6. Enjoy!

Fruit Salad

Ingredients:

- 1 lb of stemmed and quartered strawberry

- 1 Sliced banana

- 6 Blueberries

- 1 Bunch of grapes

- 2 tablespoons of sugar

- 1 Can of untrained peach slices

- 1 Can of untrained pineapple chunks

- 1 Box of dry vanilla instant pudding mix

Directions:

1. In a deep and large bowl, combine the peaches, the pineapples, and the vanilla

pudding mixture. Add the juices from the cans of the fruits

2. Combine your INGREDIENTS: very well until the pudding is completely dissolved.

3. Add the strawberries, the banana, the blueberries, the grapes, and the sugar.

4. Let the fruits salad chill; then serve and enjoy a refreshing taste!

Vegan Potato Chili Bake

Ingredients:

- 2 tsp. oregano

- Paprika to taste

- Sea salt and black pepper to taste

- ¾ cup tomato puree

- 1 cup vegetable stock

- 2 cups desired mix beans (cooked)

- 2 potato thin slices

- 1 tbsp. olive oil

- 1 tsp. garlic paste

- 1 green chili chopped

- 1 red onion chopped

- 2 carrot chopped

- 2 tsp. cumin powder

- ½ tsp. cinnamon powder

Directions:

1. Heat oil in a pan; add garlic, onion, carrot, chili and spices.
2. Mix it well cook it for 3-4 minutes.
3. Now add puree, veggie stock and beans.
4. Mix it well and cook it for additional 5 minutes.
5. Meanwhile, preheat oven to 180° C.
6. Pour this mixture in baking pan.
7. Spread layer of potato slices and bake it for 15-20 minutes.

Vegan Mutton

Ingredients:

- 1 tsp. garlic grated

- 1 tsp. ginger grated

- 1 green chili chopped

- 2 tomatoes chopped

- vegetable stock as required

- 1 cup coconut milk

- 2 tbsp. curry powder

- 2-3 cups jack fruit diced (vegan mutton)

- 2 tbsp. oil

- Handful of curry leaves

- 1 onion chopped

- Garam masala to taste

- Salt to taste

Directions:

1. Heat oil in a pan; saute ginger, garlic and onions.
2. Now add chili, curry leaves and spices.
3. Cook it for 2-3 minutes and add diced jack fruit.
4. Cook it for 5-8 minutes and then add tomatoes and stock.
5. Mix it well, cover and cook it on low for 10-15 min.
6. Now add milk and cook it for additional 5-10 min on low.
7. Then turn off the flame and garnish it with cilantro.
8. Serve hot!

Vegan Mediterranean Bowls

Ingredients:

For roasted veggies,

- 3 large-sized sweet potatoes (Diced)

- 2 and a half tablespoons of oil of your choice (Divided)

- 16 ounces/454 g of green beans (fresh or frozen, trimmed)

- 2 teaspoon of kosher salt, divided

For lemon tahini sauce,

- 3 tablespoons of lemon juice

- A quarter cup of tahini

- 3 tablespoons of water

- A quarter teaspoon of kosher salt

- Half a teaspoon of garlic powder

- Freshly ground black pepper

For assembling,

- 2 can of chickpeas, of 15 ounces/425 g

- 2 jar of marinated artichoke hearts in oil, of 6 ounces/ 170 g (Chopped)

- 2 avocado (Diced and optional)

- Three cups of arugula

Directions:

1. Heat the oven to 425 degrees Fahrenheit/220 degrees Celsius. Use parchment paper to line 3 baking sheets. In a bowl, add half a teaspoon of salt, three-quarters tablespoon of oil, and potatoes. Mix and spread over 2 baking sheet. Toss to the same bowl, half teaspoon of salt, three-quarters tablespoons

of oil, and the green beans. Spread this mixture on the other baking sheet. Place the sheets into the oven. Bake for 30 - 45 minutes. After 15 - 20 minutes, while baking, toss the veggies.

2. While the veggies are getting baked, make the lemon tahini sauce. Mix garlic powder, tahini, lemon juice, salt, and pepper. Add water and stir till a smooth mixture is formed. You can add water if required.

3. In four three-cup rectangular glasses, distribute the 3-4 artichokes, 2-third cup of chickpeas, and a handful of arugula. Then add a three-quarters cup of sweet potatoes and half a cup of roasted green beans. Drizzle lemon juice tahini sauce over this. You can use Pyrex glass containers or other containers you like for this. Add avocados only when you are about to serve. You can also add the avocado

with a bit of lemon juice the night before serving.

Tofu Stir Fry

Ingredients:

- Three cups of cauliflower rice or cooked grains

For tofu

- 2 tablespoon of coconut aminos

- 3 teaspoons of sesame oil (use a non-stick pan or use water, if you are avoiding oil)

- 2 teaspoon of chili garlic sauce

- 2 cup of extra firm tofu, pressed, cubed for crumbled

For sauce

- 3 to three tablespoons of coconut aminos or tamari

- 2 tablespoon of lime juice

- 2 tablespoon of maple syrup

- 3 tablespoons of peanut butter (Or other nut butter of your choice)

- 2 to 3 teaspoons of chili garlic sauce

To stir fry

- 2 cup of shiitake mushrooms (chopped)

- 2 cup of thinly sliced red bell pepper

- 2 cup of thinly sliced red cabbage

- 3 teaspoons of sesame oil (use water or nonstick pan, if you do not prefer oil)

- 3 cloves of garlic (Minced)

- 2 tablespoon of ginger freshly minced

- A quarter cup of green onion- thinly sliced

For Serving (optional)

- Fresh cilantro (chopped)

- Peanut sauce

- Lime wedges

- Sriracha or chili garlic sauce

Directions:

1. You need cauliflower rice to start with. Usually, leftover cauliflower rice or grains are required. If it is not ready, start cooking any grains, like quinoa, brown rice or white rice, or cauliflower rice. The time for cooking the rice or grains is not included in the Directions: time.

2. In a shallow dish, add coconut aminos, chili garlic sauce, and tofu. Toss the crumbled or cubed tofu with the other INGREDIENTS: and stir to form a coat. Let the tofu marinate.

3. In a mixing bowl, mix lime juice, maple syrup, chili garlic sauce, aminos, and peanut butter (or other nut butter, if you are using). Whisk all the INGREDIENTS: to combine perfectly. Check the taste and adjust the flavors. For more heat, add the chili garlic sauce, peanut butter for more thickness, lime juice for added acidity, and for increasing the sweetness, add maple syrup. For increased depth of flavor, add coconut aminos. Keep the bowl aside.

4. In medium-high heat, heat a skillet with rims. When heated, pour the sesame oil, or water, and add the tofu you have marinated. Cook till the tofu turns brown and flip a couple of

times for even cooking. Take off from the skillet and set aside.

5. Repeat the process of heating oil in the same high rimmed skillet, add cabbage, mushrooms, and bell pepper. Sauté the veggies and keep stirring. Place a cover on the skillet. And cook for 2-3 minutes. Stir a couple of times.

6. To this add, the green onions, ginger, and garlic. Cover with the lid after stirring, and cook for 2 or 3 minutes again.

7. Use a wooden spatula or spoon and move the veggies to 2 side of the skillet. To the other side, drop the cauliflower rice or the grains you have cooked. Cover with a lid. Cook for a couple of minutes. The contents should turn slightly brown.

8. Now take the tofu you have set aside and add this to the pan.

9. Add the sauce and stir-fry. Occasionally, toss and stir to ensure the sauce is mingled with all the INGREDIENTS:. And the contents should be hot.

10. Garnish with freshly chopped cilantro, lime wedges, chili garlic sauce, and peanut butter. You can use sriracha too.

11. Serve immediately, as it tastes good when fresh.

12. Store in an airtight container and refrigerate the leftovers. Reheat when required on the stove.

Meze Bento

Ingredients:

- 1 sliced carrot

- 2-3 readymade blossom leaves

- Handful of olives

- 1 sliced wholemeal pitta

- 2 tbsps hummus

- 4 tbsps tabbouleh

- 1 sliced baby fennel bulb

Directions:

1. Add 2 tbsp hummus in a bowl at a bento box.
2. Fill another piece together with other meze INGREDIENTS:, as stated in the list above.

Protein Patties

Ingredients:

- 2 garlic cloves, peeled, chopped

- 1 tbsp tamari

- 1 tsp dried sage

- 2 tbsps water

- 1 tsp caraway seeds

- 1 tsp turmeric

- 1 tbsp ground flax seeds

- 1 can (15 oz.) Chickpeas

- 1 tsp fennel seeds

- Pepper, salt, to taste

Directions:

1. Preheat the oven to 300f.

2. Blitz all INGREDIENTS: in a food processor until smooth and then keep aside.

3. Grease the skillet with vegetable oil and place over medium heat.

4. Add the mixture into the skillet. Shape into a patty using the back of the spoon, then season with salt, pepper, and paprika.

5. Cook for 7 minutes flip over and cook for another 7 minutes.

6. Transfer to a baking sheet and bake for 15 minutes.

7. Serve warm and enjoy.

Vegan Chickpea Pancake

Ingredients:

- ¼ cup red pepper, finely chopped

- ¼ tsp salt

- 1/8 tsp ground black pepper

- ½ cup + 2 tbsps water

- ¼ tsp garlic powder

- ¼ tsp baking powder

- 1 green onion, finely choppe d

- ½ cup chickpea flour

Directions:

1. Preheat a skillet over medium heat.

2. Mix chickpea flour, baking powder, garlic powder, pepper and salt in a bowl. Shake in the water.
3. Mix for 15 seconds, then add the onion and pepper.
4. Spray the pan with nonstick cooking spray.
5. Pour the dough and spread it. Cook for 6 minutes carefully turn to the other side and cook for 5 minutes.
6. Serve with the desired INGREDIENTS:.

Hummus Dip

Ingredients:

- 1 small clove of garlic, roughly chopped

- 1 teaspoon salt

- 1/2 teaspoon finely ground black pepper

- 1 1/2 tablespoons lemon juice (from 1/2 lemon), plus more to taste

- 1 (15-ounce) can chickpeas (roughly 2 cups drained, cooked chickpeas)

- 3 tablespoons extra-virgin olive oil

- 3 tablespoons tahini

Directions:

1. Drain and rinse the chickpeas: Drain the chickpeas into a strainer and rinse under cool running water.

2. If time and patience allows, pinch the skins from each of the chickpeas; this will make your hummus smoother.

3. Combine all INGREDIENTS: in the food processor: Combine the chickpeas, olive oil, tahini, lemon juice, garlic, salt, and pepper in the bowl of the food processor or blender.

4. Blend hummus until smooth: Process the hummus continuously until it becomes very smooth, 1 to 2 minutes.

5. Scrape down the sides of the bowl as needed to integrate any large chunks.

6. Taste and adjust seasonings: Taste and add more of any of the INGREDIENTS: to taste.

7. If your hummus is stiffer than you'd like, add more lemon juice or olive oil to thin it out and make the hummus creamier.

8. Transfer to a bowl and serve: Scrape the hummus into a bowl and serve with pita chips or raw vegetables.

9. Hummus will also keep for up to a week in a sealed container in the refrigerator.

Breaded Tofu Sticks

Ingredients:

- 14 oz extra-firm tofu

- ¼ c cornmeal

- ¼ c ground almonds or wheat flour

- salt

- pepper

- several T peanut or sesame oil

- ¼ c fine bread crumbs

Directions:

1. Drain the tofu but do not pat dry. Slice cross-wise into about 8 ½-inch slices, then once length-wise, so that you end up with about 16 equal pieces.

2. Combine cornmeal, flour, bread crumbs, salt, and pepper, and use about half of mixture to cover plate.
3. Shake excess water from tofu then place on top of dry mixture and turn to coat. Sprinkle more of the dry mixture on top as needed. Set coated pieces aside.
4. When all of the tofu is breaded, put the pan over medium heat and pour in enough oil to coat the bottom.
5. Add a single layer of tofu pieces and fry until golden, about 5 minutes. Turn and cook the second side, then repeat with remaining tofu.
6. Sprinkle with salt and serve hot.

Sweet Crepes

Ingredients:

- 1 teaspoon baking powder

- 1 tablespoon coconut sugar

- 1/8 teaspoon salt

- 1 cup of water

- 1 banana

- 1/2 cup oat flour

- 1/2 cup brown rice flour

Directions:

1. Take a blender, place all the INGREDIENTS: in it except for sugar and salt and pulse for 1 minute until smooth.

2. Take a skillet pan, place it over medium-high heat, grease it with oil and when hot, pour in ¼ cup of batter, spread it as thin as possible, and cook for 2 to 3 minutes per side until golden brown.
3. Cook remaining crepes in the same manner, then sprinkle with sugar and salt and serve.

Artichoke Quiche

Ingredients:

- 1 teaspoon minced garlic

- ¼ teaspoon salt

- ¼ teaspoon ground black pepper

- 1 teaspoon dried basil

- ½ teaspoon turmeric

- 1 tablespoon coconut oil

- 1 teaspoon Dijon mustard

- ½ cup nutritional yeast

- 14 oz tofu, soft

- 14 oz of artichokes, chopped

- 2 cups spinach

- ½ of a large onion, peeled, chopped

- 1 lemon, juiced

- 2 large tortillas, cut into half

Directions:

1. Switch on the oven, then set it to 350 degrees F and let it preheat.
2. Take a pie plate, grease it with oil, place tortilla to cover the bottom and sides of the plate and bake for 10 to 15 minutes until baked.
3. Meanwhile, take a large pan, place it over medium heat, add oil and when hot, add onion and cook for 5 minutes.
4. Then add garlic, cook for 1 minute until fragrant, stir in spinach and cook for 4 minutes until the spinach has wilted, set aside when d2.

5. Place tofu in a food processor, add all the spices, yeast, and lemon juice and pulse for 2 minutes until smooth.

6. Then add cooked onion mixture and artichokes, blend for 15 to 25 times until combined, and then pour the mixture over crust in the pie plate.

7. Bake quiche for 45 minutes until d2, then cut it into wedges and serve.

Keto Fried Chicken

Ingredients:

- 2 packs Pork crackling

- 1 tbsp Garlic powder

- ½ tbsp Smoked Paprika

- 100 ml Double cream

- Salt & Pepper to taste

- 6 Skin on chicken breasts

- 2 Large free-range eggs

- 175g Almond flour

- 100 g Parmesan or hard cheese (grated)

Directions:

1. Preheat oven to 200$_0$C and line a large baking sheet with parchment paper.
2. Pat each chicken breast dry with paper towels.
3. Season with a pinch of salt and pepper on each side. Wash your hands after handling raw meat.
4. In a mixing bowl, whish together the eggs and double cream.
5. Using a shallow bowl, mix the flour, crushed pork crackling, parmesan, garlic powder and paprika.
6. Add a pinch of salt and pepper.
7. Dip an individual chicken breast into the egg mixture to fully coat.
8. Shake off any drips and then press into the flour coating mixture to fully cover.
9. Place on the baking sheet. Repeat for all breasts.

10. Bake the chicken in the centre of the oven for around 45 minutes.

11. The chicken is cooked when it is no longer pink in the middle.

Dressed Broccoli Salad

Ingredients:

- 3 Heads broccoli cut into florets

- 100 g Cheddar (grated)

- 1 Small red onion (halved and sliced)

- 50 g Toasted sliced almonds

- 4 Rashers smoked back bacon (crisped and crumbled)

- 2 tbsp freshly chopped chives

- 65 g Mayonnaise

- 3 tbsp Apple cider vinegar

- 1 tbsp Dijon mustard

- Salt & Pepper to taste

Directions:

1. Using the medium saucepan, boil 1.5 litres of water with 6 pinches of salt. Prepare the mixing bowl with cold water and plenty of ice.

2. Add the broccoli florets to the boiling water and cook until tender, 1-2 minutes. Remove these from the saucepan with a slotted spoon and immediately chill in the ice water. When cool, drain all the florets with a colander.

3. Mix the mayonnaise, vinegar and mustard together in a small bowl to create a dressing with a whisk. Watch the sugar levels.

4. Combine all the salad INGREDIENTS: in a large bowl with the dressing and toss. Refrigerate until ready to serve.

Mouth-Watering Basil, Tomato & Mushroom Omelets

Ingredients:

- 1 Tablespoon of unsalted butter

- 2 Tablespoons of low fat cream cheese

- 1 Tablespoon of basil leaves finely chopped

- 2 tomatoes cut in half

- 3 medium eggs

- 1 Tablespoon of snipped chives

- 1 ⅓ cup sliced chestnut mushrooms

Directions:

1. Preheat the grill to 400 degrees F.

2. Place the tomatoes on a baking tray and grill for 10 minutes or until the tomatoes are scorched, turning occasionally.
3. Take the tomatoes out of the grill and release the juice by squashing them slightly.
4. In a small bowl, whisk the eggs, add the chives and continue to whisk.
5. Heat the butter in a large frying pan, add the mushrooms and cook for 8 minutes or until they become tender.
6. Remove the mushrooms from the pan and set to 2 side.
7. Pour the eggs into the frying pan and fry until it sets on the bottom.
8. Spoon the mushrooms onto 2 side of the omelets.
9. Top with the basil leaves and the cream cheese.
10. Flip the omelets and then place in the grill to cook for 2 minutes.

11. Once cooked, transfer onto a plate and serve with the tomatoes on the side.

Wonderful Waffles Multi Grain Style

Ingredients:

- 1 teaspoon of baking powder

- 1 teaspoon of baking soda

- 1 teaspoon of ground cinnamon

- 2 medium eggs

- ¼ cup of packed brown sugar

- 1 Tablespoon of olive oil

- 1 teaspoon of vanilla extract

- 2 cups of buttermilk

- ½ cup of rolled oats

- ⅔ cup of whole wheat flour

- ¼ cup of cornmeal

Directions:

1. In a medium sized bowl, mix together the oats and the buttermilk and allow it to sit for 15 minutes.
2. In a large bowl, whisk the cinnamon, salt, baking soda, baking powder, cornmeal, all-purpose flour, and whole wheat flour.
3. Add the vanilla, oil, sugar and eggs into the oat mixture and stir together thoroughly.
4. Spray a waffle iron with cooking oil and heat it.
5. Spoon the batter into the waffle iron so that three fourths of the surface is covered.

6. Cook for 5 minutes until the waffles are golden brown and crisp. Repeat with the rest of the batter.

Potato Leek Soup

Ingredients:

- 1 teaspoon of black pepper

- 2 teaspoons of celery salt

- 2 carrots, sliced

- 2 teaspoons of sea salt

- 1 small onion, diced

- 4 cups of vegetable broth

- 3-4 small or medium potatoes

- 2 large leeks, sliced in 2-inch pieces (washed and rinsed)

Directions:

1. In a large cooking pot, pour in the vegetable broth and bring to a boil on medium-high.

2. Wash, scrub and sliced the potatoes (removing the skins or leaving them attached) and add to the broth.

3. Add in the celery salt, carrots, sea salt, onion, and black pepper and continue to cook on medium until potatoes are tender.

4. Remove the pot from the stove and allow to cool.

5. Process in batches in a food processor or blender, until the soup, is smooth and creamy.

6. Return to the large pot and reheat, then stir in the leaks.

7. Serve with a dollop of vegan sour cream and meatless bacon bits.

8. If leek is not in season and you'd like to make this soup, try substituting green onion or fresh dill instead.

9. Creamy potato soup can be modified for many other INGREDIENTS:, including chopped

spinach, slices of smoked tofu or Tempe and parsley.

Tomato Sauce With Spaghetti

Ingredients:

- 1 teaspoon of chili powder

- 1 teaspoon of black pepper

- 2 cloves of garlic, crushed

- 1 small onion, diced

- ½ package of spaghetti noodles

- 1 block of tempeh (plain, unflavored)

- 1 large can of pureed tomatoes

- 2 tablespoons of oregano

- 1 tablespoon of thyme

Directions:

1. In a small skillet, heat the olive oil and combine the onion and garlic.

2. Sauté for a few minutes and add in the marinated tempeh and ½ cup of the tomato sauce.

3. Reduce heat and simmer for 8-10 minutes, then remove. In a large cooking pot, pour the contents of the skillet with the remainder of the tomato sauce.

4. Heat and stir slowly on medium, though avoid bringing to a boil.

5. Stir in the oregano, thyme, chili powder, black pepper, and salt.

6. Blend and cook for another 15-20 minutes. Prepare the spaghetti by boiling 3-4 cups of water in a second cooking pot and add sea salt.

7. Add the spaghetti and cook until tender, then drain and rinse.

8. Serve the tempeh and tomato sauce over the noodles and top with vegan parmesan or garnish with fresh parsley.

Roasted Root Vegetables In A Miso Sauce

Ingredients:

- 2 medium yams, sliced into large chunks (quarters)

- 1 small rutabaga, sliced into quarters

- 1 beet, sliced into 2-inch-thick slices

- Fresh parsley to garnish

- 2 large carrots, peeled and sliced lengthwise

- 2-3 parsnips, peeled and sliced lengthwise

- 1 cup of radishes, washed, scrubbed and stems removed

Miso sauce:

- 1 cup of vegetable broth

- 1 teaspoon of soy sauce

- 1 tablespoon of miso paste

Directions:

1. To prepare the vegetables, preheat the oven to 350 degrees and grease a deep baking dish lightly with olive oil.
2. Add all the vegetables to the pan and set aside. In a saucepan, add the vegetable broth and bring to a boil, then stir in the miso paste and soy sauce, whisking while reducing heat to low to simmer.
3. Pour half of the miso sauce over the vegetables, then place in the oven and bake for 30-40 minutes, or until all vegetables are tender, then pour the remaining sauce on the vegetables, and cook for another 15-20 minutes, then remove and cool slightly before serving with parsley.

Apple And Sweet Potato Latkes With Tahiti Sauce

Ingredients:

- Spelt flour 2 tablespoons

- Olive oil 1 tablespoon

- Turmeric 1 teaspoon

- Pepper to taste

- Kale for garnish

- Sweet Potato 1 large, peeled

- Apple 1, peeled and quartered

- Onion ½, diced

- Salt 1 teaspoon

- Arrowroot powder 1 tablespoon

Tahini sauce

- Tahini 3 tablespoons

- Juice of 2 lemon

- Maple syrup 1 tablespoon

- Water as needed

- Squirt of Sriracha

Directions:

1. To make the sauce, in a bowl, combine all the INGREDIENTS: and whisk together. Set aside.

2. Into a large mixing bowl, grate the sweet potato and the apple. Squeeze as much liquid out of the grated apple and potato and transfer the squeezed mixture into another bowl.

3. Add the pepper, turmeric, olive oil, spelt flour, arrowroot, onion, and salt. Mix to combine.

4. Heat a skillet over medium-high heat. Add 2 tablespoons of olive oil. Take about ¼ cup of the latke batter in your hand and squeeze it together to make a flat round patty.
5. Place the patty on the hot pan and use a spatula to press down. Cook until golden brown and crispy, about 2 to 4 minutes per side.
6. Transfer to a plate cover with paper towel to cool.
7. Repeat with the remaining batter.
8. Serve with sauce.

Vegan Omelet

Ingredients:

- Black pepper 1/8

- Ener-G Egg Replacer ½ teaspoon

- Water ¼ cup + 1 tablespoon

- Any leafy green 1 handful, torn with hands

- Any veggie or filling of your choice

- Toppings parsley, hot sauce, ketchup, salsa

- Chickpea flour ¼ cup

- Nutritional yeast 1 tablespoon

- Baking powder ½ teaspoon

- Turmeric ¼ teaspoon

- Chopped chives ½ teaspoon

- Garlic powder ¼ teaspoon

Directions:

1. Except for the greens and optional veggies, mix all INGREDIENTS: in a small bowl.
2. Let stand for 5 minutes, and add more water if too thick. The batter should be pancake batter consistency.
3. Meanwhile, oil a non-stick pan and heat over medium heat. Pour the batter into the hot pan like you are making a pancake. Cover the pan with a lid and cook on low heat until bubbles form the surface and edge dry out for about 3 minutes.
4. Now add the veggies and greens to 2-half of the omelette and with a spatula, fold the omelette over in half and cook for 2 more minutes, uncovered.
5. Remove and place on a plate. Top with hot sauce, ketchup, and salsa.

www.ingramcontent.com/pod-product-compliance
Lightning Source LLC
Chambersburg PA
CBHW060504030426
42337CB00015B/1736